THE CAUSE OF THE OBESITY EPIDEMIC

By John McKenna BA. MB. ChB.

Copyright © John Mckenna November 2012

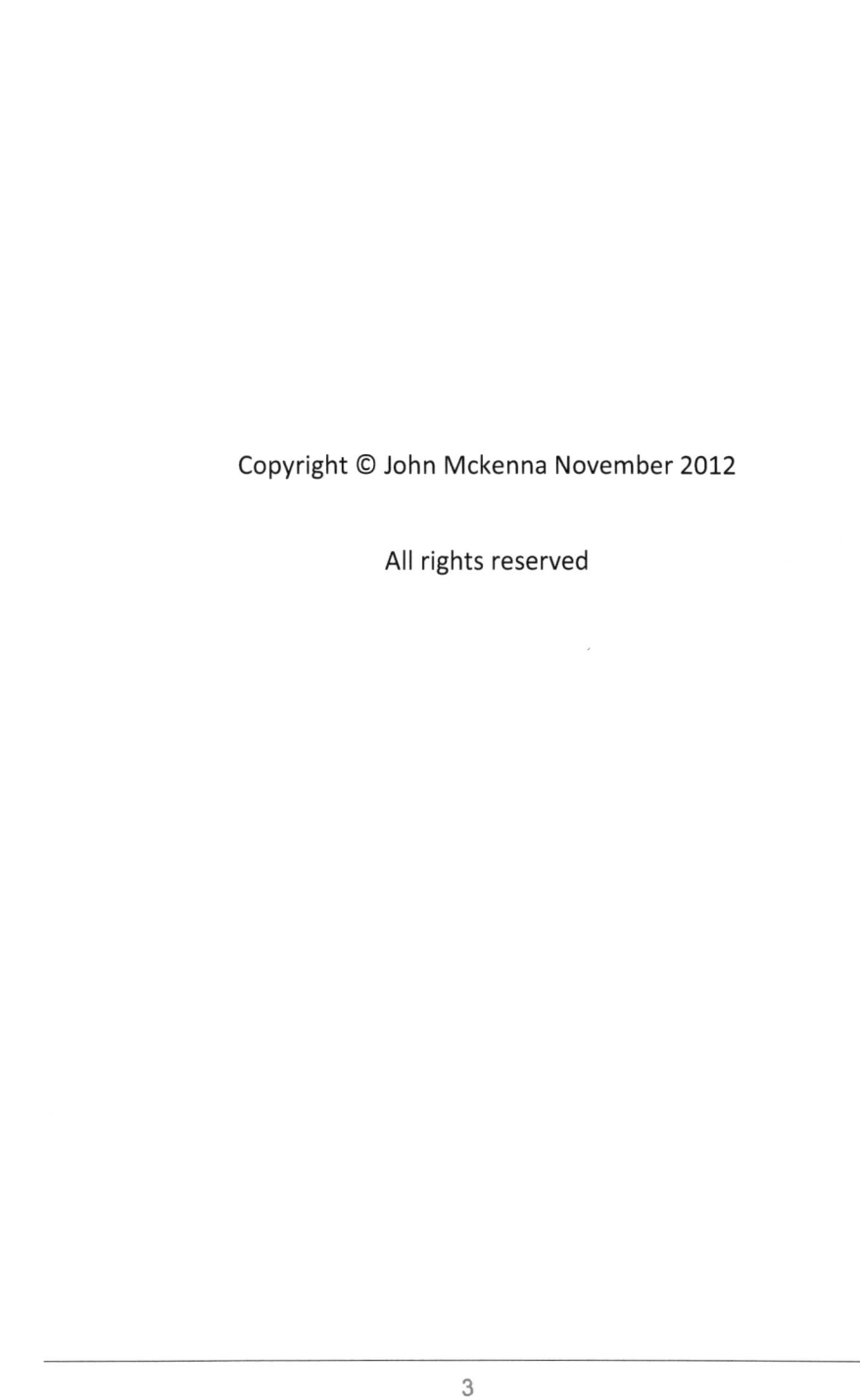

All rights reserved

Table of contents

Introduction

Chapter 1 - The Problem

Chapter 2 - The Human Factor

Chapter 3 - What Changed to Cause this Epidemic?

Chapter 4 - The Food Pyramid

Chapter 5 - Sugar Is Toxic

Chapter 6 - Effects of High Uric Acid Levels

Chapter 7 - Effects of Fructose on the Brain

Chapter 8 - Fructose is Dangerous

Chapter 9 - Why the Silence?

Chapter 10 – The Role of Emotions in Gastrointestinal Illness

Chapter 11 – The Treatment of Obesity

Chapter 12 – Weight Loss Supplements

Conclusion

Acknowledgements

Bibliography

Introduction

Having spent nine years in university studying science and then medicine, I was shocked to hear the nutritional advice being given to people to help them lose weight. It is, in plain language, the wrong advice. For example, the advice to 'eat more carbohydrates and less fat' is not only wrong, but is bad for your general health. Also, exercise makes you feel better and is good for your general health but does not contribute significantly to weight loss. Worse still, something happened to our food in the mid-1970s to begin the obesity epidemic, and strangely nobody wants to speak about it; it's a big secret, a big fat secret. The purpose of this book is to expose this secret and give you the information you need to help protect your own health, and that of your family. This book will tell you the truth!

I have spent the last twenty five years treating children with recurrent infections, which led to the publication of my first book "Alternatives to Antibiotics" (Gill & MacMillan 1992) and treating digestive problems in adults which led to the publication of "Hard to Stomach" (Gill & Macmillan

2002) both of which have been best sellers. I use nutrition to help solve medical problems and try to get people off conventional medicine where possible. With this in mind I have set up "The Food Clinic" to not only help people lose weight but also to continue to solve problems through diet, nutritional supplements and emotional healing. What has become apparent to me over the years, and especially in treating gut problems, is that buried emotions play a big role in our ill health, especially weight gain. This is why I asked my good friend and colleague, Dr Pradeep Chadha, to write one chapter in this book, and to assist in the work of The Food Clinic, as I believe a combination of diet, nutritional supplements and emotional healing can bring all of us great rewards.

I hope this book is helpful to you. Wishing you good health.

John Mckenna. BA, MB.ChB.

The Food Clinic, Edgewater, Killincooley Beg, Kilmuckridge, Co Wexford, Ireland - E-mail: mckennaje@gmail.com

Chapter 1- The Problem

There is a solution to the scourge of obesity. Before rushing straight to the solution, however, it is necessary to explore the topic in a bit more depth so that you will be able to better understand what I will be discussing, and be able to see the simple, logical arguments presented here. We first must appreciate the true extent of this epidemic and how it affects each of us individually, while simultaneously learning something about how we got into this state within such a short space of time—a little over three decades. In my explanations, I will cut out as much of the medical and scientific jargon as possible and try to paint as straightforward a picture as I can.

All of us are aware that, as a nation, we are more overweight than we were thirty years ago. Yet, how common are the conditions of being overweight, having obesity, and having morbid obesity in our society? How many adults walking the street do you think are overweight in England? How many adults do you think are obese? How many boys between the ages of two and fifteen would you say are obese? What about for girls? How many children are predicted to be overweight by the year 2050 in the UK? What do these terms mean, exactly? I will define them in a moment.

In England, sixty-six out of one hundred adults are presently overweight—that's two-thirds of the population. As we progress through this epidemic, two things are becoming apparent:

a) More and more people are being affected.

b) Those who are overweight find that their weight increases faster with time. Obesity and morbid obesity develops more quickly with time if individuals go without treatment.

So—to put simply—more of us are getting fat, and the fat are getting fatter, faster. Clearly, this is not a story of putting on a few extra pounds and having difficulty losing it. This is a more serious situation in which virtually a whole nation is changing into obese and morbidly obese people. It is a story of the total breakdown of the normal weight-control mechanisms in the body. This, in turn, leads to a whole host of medical problems that I will describe in the coming chapters. The epidemic weight gain of the nation resembles a horror story depicting how a nation can be destroyed. It's not affecting just America and the UK—it's affecting most countries with populations that eat modern, processed foods.

Japan, for example, used to have a very healthy diet and population until very recently. Today, they are performing bariatric surgery (in which the size of the stomach is reduced) on children because of their obesity. In the UK, of the sixty-six percent (66%) of the population who are overweight, twenty-five percent (25%) of them are obese. Of these twenty-five percent (25%), many have type 2 diabetes, hypertension, abnormal cholesterol levels, gout, and heart disease. If they don't already have these, they are at an increased risk of developing one or more of these disorders. So as time progresses and 2011 transitions into 2012, the figures of sixty-six percent (66%) and twenty-five percent (25%) continue to rise as more of us become victims. Greater numbers of people are finding themselves ill and dependent on drugs to live a normal life.

Now to the children—what percentage did you guess were obese? The percentage of obesity in children matches that of adults. Nineteen percent (19%) of boys and fifteen percent (15%) of girls are obese as of 2010, but this figure is rising rapidly. It is rising so fast that by the year 2050, there are estimates that ninety percent (90%) of children will be overweight or obese. This staggering number includes almost all of the population's children. It seems hard to believe—as if it's an idea out of the realms of science fiction. In case you find this questionable, here are the UK's World Health Organisation statistics for the period 1966 – 1999:

TABLE 1:

Percentage of men in each BMI category (UK):

Men	1966	1972	1982	1989	1999
BMI <18.5	2.3	1.9	1.3	0.6	0.3
BMI 18.5-24.9	83.7	72.6	54.7	44	27.9
BMI 25 -29.9	12.8	23.0	37.8	44.7	49.2
BMI >30	1.2	2.7	6.2	10.6	22.6

TABLE 2

Percentage of women in each BMI category (UK):

Women	1966	1972	1982	1989	1999
BMI <18.5	7.8	5.4	3.7	1.6	0.3
BMI 18.5-24.9	81.1	78.0	70.4	58.5	37.6
BMI 25-29.9	9.2	13.9	19.0	25.8	36.3
BMI >30	1.8	2.7	6.9	14.0	25.8

Look at these figures closely. In Table 1, the percentage of men with normal weight, or rather normal BMI (18.5 – 24.9), dropped from eighty-three percent (83%) to twenty-seven percent (27%) between 1966 and 1999. In other words, there are fewer men with a healthy BMI as time progresses. The number of obese men rose from one point two percent (1.2%) to twenty-two point six percent (22.6%) in the space of thirty-three years.

In the USA, the figures are slightly worse than the rest of the world. Seventy percent (70%) of Americans are now overweight or obese. Every country has always had a small percentage of overweight people, but this big change in the statistics began in the mid-'70s to early '80s.

Something happened in the mid-'70s to explain this sudden change of events. Can you guess what changed? Hold your guess for a moment while we go through the task of defining the terms, as promised earlier. These definitions help to clarify terms such as BMI, overweight, obesity, morbid obesity, etc.

Let's start with the term BMI, which replaced the term 'weight for height' some years ago. BMI stands for body mass index. It is defined as your weight in kilograms divided by your height squared in meters squared. So, if your weight is 70 kg (Mr. Average), and your height is 1.8 meters, your BMI would be calculated as:

70 / 1.8 x 1.8 = 70 / 3.24 = 21.8, approximately.

BMI measurements are placed in different categories so that doctors and scientists know if you are underweight, overweight, or a normal and healthy weight. Here are the five main categories of BMI:

<18.5 is underweight

18.5 – 24.9 is normal

25 – 29.9 is overweight

30 -39.9 is obese

> 40 is morbid obesity

We believe BMI is supposed to tell us if we are fat, and if so, how fat. But does it? Actually no, it doesn't. It tells us when we are carrying a lot of weight for our height, but it does not tell us if the extra weight is due to fat or to protein (as with body builders, rugby players, etcetera). BMI is still just a measure of 'weight for height' and it would be a lot simpler if they continued to refer to it in those terms. I guess scientists like the more complicated term, BMI.

The BMI measurement also does not tell us where one has gained or lost weight. It is helpful to know if the weight gain is central (around the waist), as this is a clear sign of obesity. Waist circumference can be measured by using an old-fashioned tape measure.

Armed with your BMI and waist circumference, you can then see how you measure up to the rest of the population and which of the above categories you fit into. If you never have had your BMI and waist circumference measured, don't bother just now. Read this book first, and then decide. Due to our statistics, it is a reasonable guess that your weight is increasing and that you are progressing along the road towards obesity. The road looks like this:

Normal weight -------> Overweight -------> Obese

If you are already obese, most doctors will have two objectives in treatment; neither of which involves moving you backwards along this road. They will aim to delay or prevent the onset of hypertension, diabetes, heart disease, and abnormal blood cholesterol by the use of drugs. Secondly, they will try to halt the progression of your weight gain by holding the weight constant. Lowering your overall weight permanently is quite hard to achieve, so it's not their objective. Most obese people who do manage to lose weight will inevitably put it back on again, as they have not been educated about the real cause of weight gain. This is part of the reason that doctors stick to the two main objectives mentioned above.

However, this is classic negative thinking on the part of western medicine. You have the choice to accept this negative approach or reject it. You must make this choice. Do you genuinely believe there is an answer to the obesity riddle? Or do you believe there is no answer and that eventually most people will end up obese?

Look at it this way: if the problem began in the mid-'70s and there was no evidence of an obesity epidemic prior to that, it should be possible to discover what went wrong, reverse it, and get almost everyone's weight back to the normal weight range. That's what I aim to show you in this book. So do not despair, as there is most definitely an answer which you are about to discover.

In order to find a credible solution to the obesity problem, the solution must meet the following criteria:

- It must explain why the epidemic began in the mid-'70s in the US, and a little later in the UK.

- It must explain why all ages are being affected—even young children and infants.

- It must be an environmental factor and not genetic, as the gene pool did not alter suddenly in the 1970s. (Unless, of course, little green aliens came and altered our DNA.)

- It must explain why many obese people also have a range of medical conditions, such as type 2 diabetes, hypertension, etc.

- It must explain why obesity is now a global phenomenon.

- It must explain why the poor tend to be the most affected in many countries.

The aim of this book is to explain all of the above convincingly so that you will be left without any doubt about the true cause of this epidemic.

Finally, let's peek into the future: by 2015, the World Health Organisation predicts that 2.3 billion people in the world will be overweight and 700 million of these people will be obese. We have already surpassed all previous predictions, so it may be safe to increase these numbers a bit. They also predict that by 2050, ninety percent (90%) of children will be overweight.

It's best to read that last sentence again. Yes, it is true and very shocking! To me, the future looks quite bleak if we continue with the present paradigm that overeating and lack of exercise cause obesity. For this, the mainstay of treatment is eat less and exercise more. If this was correct, the epidemic would show signs of coming under control. Rather, it is getting worse as these predictions testify. The future is not bleak if there is a credible scientific answer. Fortunately, there is one and so we can all start to reverse this trend. There is a way out of this impasse.

So what exactly is our challenge here? Obesity is a major epidemic; it is global and affects all age groups. It began about thirty years ago and continues unabated. To date, no one has found a concrete cause and, therefore, no treatment has been proven to work permanently.

Chapter 2 - The Human Factor

Here we are going to look at a few of the many problems suffered by obese people. These physical and mental problems are a direct result of being overweight and, for the most part, were not there prior to a rise in BMI.

These problems are not the individual's fault. It is their environment—and in particular their diet—that is creating the problem. You may believe that we 'create' our own diets, and while it's true that we do have a certain amount of choice in our diets, it is also true that we are limited by what is actually available. That limitation increases in direct proportion to the level of poverty of the person in question. Even if you were quite wealthy, it would not be practical to pay inflated prices or drive long distances to purchase healthier food if cheaper, pre-cooked/ pre-prepared food is available locally.

Many members of society perceive obese people as alien, lazy, and the cause of their own misfortune—this includes members of the health professions as well. Many doctors, nurses, public health officials, and dieticians think of obesity as a self-inflicted condition. It is the lack of knowledge of these professionals that is at fault. Obese and overweight people are victims of this ignorance and perceptions and are mostly blameless. It is ridiculous to think that so many people would actually choose to be obese. It is even more ridiculous to think that innocent children—including infants—choose to be obese, or that their parents would choose this lifestyle for them.

Case History

James: BMI 32

James was a twenty-seven year-old man who came to ask for help with his sleep problems and his overactive gut. He had been diagnosed with type 2 diabetes and was on medication to control his blood sugar level. He told me that he had an insatiable appetite and never felt full. He was eating mostly burgers, fried chips, bread, and pizza to fill him. He also drank lots of soft drinks, fruit juice, and water. He had recently been diagnosed with high blood pressure and was taking medication for that as well.

His doctor advised him to try eating less and to exercise twice a day, every day. He referred him to a dietician for advice. The dietician recommended that he eat more fruit, vegetables, lean protein, and low fat dairy such as low-fat cheese and skimmed milk. James found it easy to exercise by playing tennis because he had always loved the game, but he found it difficult to follow the dietary advice since the extra exercise only increased his hunger pangs. He described himself as being addicted to carbohydrates, and he had no taste for fruit, vegetables, or any of those other foods. He just craved more and more starchy foods and soft drinks. When he did not consume them, he immediately began to feel withdrawal symptoms: cravings, depression, and irritability. Eventually he gave in and ate starch, but then it quickly escalated to binge eating as his withdrawal symptoms decreased with consumption. He felt trapped in this cycle of addiction and his doctor and dietician were not able to help him escape it. Every day was a huge battle for James as his weight kept increasing despite trying to follow his doctor's advice.

Recently, he had begun to have sleeping problems; his partner told him he was snoring, mouth breathing, and had sleep apnea (temporarily stopping breathing while asleep) on occasion. This is what brought him to see me. I explained to him that I had to treat the root cause of his obesity as this was producing all of his other health problems. In other words, certain substances in his diet were causing him to put on weight, which blocked certain hormones from functioning and induced all of his other difficulties. When he finally grasped what was wrong with his body's biochemistry, James realized what he had to do to fix it. Between the two of us, we managed to not only get him off all medications, but to also decrease his BMI and ultimately return to a normal, healthy weight.

James's story is very typical. For some people, the advice to eat less and exercise more does work in the short term. Unless the person has amazing willpower, however, hunger takes over and the person cannot maintain the program of treatment, and so a vicious cycle of dieting and binging commences.

We are thirty years into this epidemic and it is clear that conventional medical advice is not working as the overweight are becoming obese, the obese are becoming morbidly obese, and more of the human population are joining this weight gain race. Telling people to exercise more simply does not work. There is not a scrap of hard scientific evidence to suggest that it may be helpful.[DL6] Exercise is generally good for everyone, but it's not the solution to the problem at hand.

Telling someone to eat less also does not make sense for someone with an insatiable appetite. Would it not be wiser to find the cause of this uncontrollable appetite and fix that? Wisdom is unfortunately lacking. Shortly, I will explain the hormonal problem causing this insatiable appetite and will show you what you need to do in order to correct it.

Chapter 3 - What Changed to Cause this Epidemic?

The situation notably worsened on planet Earth just over thirty years ago. Two significant events happened in the US during the mid-70s. First came the announcement from a senate committee, the Surgeon General's office, the American Heart Association, and a variety of other sources that animal fat was implicated in heart disease and that everyone should reduce their intake of these fats. This led to a growth in the development of low-fat foods.

Then came the food pyramid to reinforce this message. People were told to eat less fat and to eat more carbohydrates. They advised this because, apparently, there was adequate scientific evidence that 'proved' animal fat was poor for your health. The primary source of this evidence was a study published in the medical journal, Circulation, in 1970 by Professor Ancel Keys (University of Minnesota). It was entitled "Coronary Heart Disease in Seven Countries" and was published in seven volumes—a massive study.

This study began in 1956 with an annual budget of $200,000—a large sum of money in those days. It involved investigating potential risk factors for heart disease among males in seven countries—Finland, Holland, USA, Italy, Greece, Yugoslavia, and Japan. These men were followed up by researchers every five years to track how many had died of heart disease, and then were analysed to find the potential risk factors. Keys's intention was to prove an association between the intake of animal fat and cholesterol levels in the bloodstream, and to prove an association between cholesterol levels and heart disease.

His findings suggested the following:

a) There is no relationship between cigarette smoking and heart disease.

b) There is no relationship between lack of exercise and heart disease.

c) There is no relationship between body weight (BMI) and heart disease.

d) There is some weak relationship between high blood pressure and heart disease.

e) There is a definite relationship between blood cholesterol level and heart disease.

f) There is a definite relationship between dietary intake of animal fat and blood cholesterol.

None of his findings are actually correct considering what we know today, but the idea that fats were possibly playing a role as a risk factor became ingrained in the minds of people. This idea also influenced opinions and advice given by doctors and the government. Years later, Ancel Keys himself admitted that dietary fat did not play a role in heart disease ("The Soft Science of Fat" Science March 30 2001).

There has been major criticisms of this study over the years. The main criticisms are as followed:

- He hand-picked the seven countries (which introduces bias).

- He excluded women from his study.

- He admitted that there was insufficient evidence to draw meaningful conclusions.

- It was an epidemiological study based on statistics.

- The data had not been analysed correctly.

Don't worry if you find the terminology challenging. Basically, it implies that the whole study—despite being very expensive—was biased and therefore invalid from the outset. Yet it is still quoted as the primary evidence in favour of restricting fats in the diet.

The Framington Heart Study is another bit of evidence in favour of a low-fat diet. This study, which also looks at risk factors of heart disease, began in 1948 and is still on-going today. In 1961, this study suggested a link between raised LDL cholesterol (so called 'bad cholesterol') and heart disease (coronary artery disease). This confirmed Ancel Keys's finding, and so Keys made the cover of Time magazine and hailed the birth of the anti-fat movement.

The lead researcher of the Framington Heart Study later admitted that there was no suggestion of a link between dietary animal fat and heart disease. If you are confused right now, you are not alone. Everyone in the field, including the researchers, is permanently confused. In fact, wading through all the research that has been compiled up to date will likely leave you fit for the lunatic asylum.

The long and short of it is that there is no evidence linking animal fat with heart disease. Despite that, the low-fat idea has become part of governmental and medical thinking.

Senator George McGovern, who chaired the Select Committee on Nutrition & Human Needs for a nine-year period, came to the conclusion in 1977 that it was prudent to endorse a nationwide low-fat diet. His findings angered many of the scientists and doctors working in this field of study. His conclusions were proven incorrect by the early 1980s when four clinical trials all revealed that dietary fat had no effect whatsoever on heart disease. However, it was too late; the horse had bolted.

Senator McGovern's report had already resulted in many government departments advising people to lower animal fat in the diet. To add insult to injury, the Surgeon General's Office spent eleven years (1988-1999) examining all of the research and trying to validate the low-fat message which had already been broadcasted to the nation. They could not validate it. One might have expected a public apology, a reversal of the message, and a few rolling heads. Nothing was said, no heads rolled, and the gospel according to Senator McGovern is still being preached. Why? There is no solid scientific evidence to back up the low-fat theory (or its gospel). There is, however, a lot of evidence suggesting a link between a high-carbohydrate diet and heart disease.

There is also evidence linking certain carbohydrates to obesity and all of the disorders that obese people suffer from—i.e. high blood pressure, gout, abnormal blood cholesterol (raised LDL and low HDL), and type 2 diabetes. Hold on to that idea while we explore what else happened in the mid-70s.

The second major catastrophe to come out of America happened during 1975 in the food processing industry. In a political effort to sell cheaper food, and because the National Institute for Health was advocating a high-carbohydrate/low-fat diet, a cheap method of producing low-fat food—which is generally unpalatable—taste better was introduced by the food chemists of the major food manufacturers. It was called High Fructose Corn Syrup and was abbreviated to HFCS. It is made from genetically modified corn and has a high concentration of fructose, which is much sweeter than glucose. It was so cheap and was so sweet that it became an immediate success. It became so successful that today almost every processed food has it as an ingredient.

This ingredient is classified under various names such as fructose, fructose-glucose, corn syrup, and HFCS. It is the low-cost, long shelf life alternative to animal fat. In reality, it is a mixture of fructose and glucose. As we will see shortly, this is a particularly dangerous combination of sugars—especially if consumed in excessive quantities. Fructose is the most fattening carbohydrate of them all.

The mid-70s in the USA were quite eventful. They actually changed the course of human health. They witnessed both the introductions of the low-fat diet and HFCS as a sweetener. Both of these factors arrived at the same time to form a true weapon of mass destruction (WMD). There is no need to search in Iraq for WMDs when they are sitting in your cupboard at home. HFCS is in ordinary foods such as factory-produced breads, hamburger buns, hot dog buns, biscuits, cakes, waffles, tomato ketchup, soft drinks, sports drinks, chocolates, and many other foods. If you check your cupboards, you will see this for yourself. You will probably be shocked by how many products contain it. Even flavoured milks and many fruit juices have HFCS. You are eating more HFCS by eating fast foods since the dastardly ingredient is prevalent in many buns, burgers, sauces, dips, soft drinks, and desserts.

The food chemists who added this cheap sweetener to the food chain were fully aware of the consequences to their actions. By 1971 it was well known what the dangers of high amounts of fructose were. Obesity was the principal danger. Before going on to discuss the effects of HFCS on the body, I would like us to look first at something called the food pyramid.

Chapter 4 - The Food Pyramid

I'm sure you have seen the food pyramid produced by the US government in 1992. If not, check it out on the website www.cnpp.usda.gov Do you understand what it means? What is a serving of grain? Try explaining the pyramid to a relative or friend and see how far you get.

This is another product of the USA. It is not the first food pyramid ever produced, but it is the first to have such a profound effect on the American nation. Also, because many other countries have copied the USA model, it has influenced other nations as well. It was produced by the United States Department of Agriculture (USDA) to advise Americans what to eat. Despite lacking any valid scientific evidence, the USDA saw fit to tell the nation, and indirectly the rest of the world as well, to increase our carbohydrate intake and to reduce our intake of animal fat. Shortly afterwards, many other countries followed suit and produced their own version (including Ireland and Great Britain).

I'm sure you have seen these pyramids as they're in many public places: school classrooms, hospitals, doctor's waiting rooms, school and university textbooks, and many other places. The message conveyed in the pyramid is to use fats sparingly and to eat lots of carbohydrates. This message is an insult to our health, since it is common knowledge that too many carbohydrates make you fat. My mother knew this, as I'm sure yours did as well. The whole world knows this. Strangely, the employees of the USDA don't seem to.

Secondly, the pyramid is advocating that you use fats, especially animal fats, sparingly. Again, this is an insult to one's instinct and intelligence. I grew up on raw eggs, whole milk, butter, cheese, lard, yoghurt, fatty meats, oily fish, butter on potatoes and on vegetables, etcetera. This message is implying that my mother, my grandmother, and all the generations before her were wrong—basically everyone who has walked this planet prior to 1992. Some cultures such as the Masai in East Africa live solely on cow's milk, meat, and blood—which are all full of animal fats. The Eskimo, Sami, Fulani, and more all base their diets on animal produce. According to the USDA, they are all fools and unhealthy in the eyes of the USDA.

Why try to convey such a message? The USDA has nothing to do with human health at all, and has no business advising anyone about diet. The USDA is there to promote the food industry, especially American food manufacturers. Yes, the USDA is promoting the very companies that incorporate HFCS into modern processed foods. I smell vested interests at work here—what about you? Why did the National Institute of Health, the Surgeon General's Office, the American Medical Association, or the American Dietetic Association not produce this food pyramid? Maybe they wouldn't have agreed with it. Maybe they didn't have such a cozy relationship with the food manufacturers. Remember that these companies are motivated by their ability to make a lot of money by convincing us to minimise the intake of God-given food in favour of man-made food. This reminds me of a wise quote from Barry Groves: "Man is the only species clever enough to make his own food and stupid enough to eat it."

To explain the absolute importance of animal fat, I have to explain some simple biology: A human cell, such as a skin cell, is surrounded by a cell membrane which controls what enters and leaves the cell. This cell membrane is composed of mostly animal fat and cholesterol—the two foods we are told to reduce in our diet

The cell membrane is also composed of protein. Inside the cell are membranes surrounding the different parts of the cell. For example, the nucleus that contains the chromosomes (the genetic material) has a nuclear membrane, and the mitochondria have membranes as well so that each part of the cell is separate from the other parts. All of these membranes are composed of the same materials: fat and protein. The structural integrity of a cell therefore depends on fat and protein. These two foods are essential for growing children, especially since they are building new cells all of the time. They are essential for everyone, however, regardless of age. The healthiest people on the planet eat mainly animal fat and protein. You cannot survive without fat or protein, but you can without carbohydrates.

Animal fat is also called saturated fat. Of all the fats and oils created by nature or animal, saturated fat is the only one that is a solid. Compare butter and olive oil, for example. Butter (saturated) is solid at room temperature while olive oil (unsaturated) is liquid. Animal fat's solidity gives the membrane structural integrity; you could not build good membranes using unsaturated fats such as olive oil. Because of this, it is critically important to eat lots of saturated fats such as butter, cheese, and whole milk.

Saturated fats are also very important because they contain fat-soluble vitamins—vitamin A, D, E, and K. These vitamins are essential for good health. Vitamin A has many functions in the body, but it is best known for its role in vision or eyesight. In fact, our eyes contain an abundance of vitamin A and this is why isolated people often eat the eyes of animals. Vitamin D facilitates the absorption of calcium and phosphorus to make strong bones and teeth. Many people with osteoporosis take calcium supplements. These is no point in doing this unless you consume a lot of animal fat at the same time; if you consume low-fat options you will not be able to absorb much of the calcium. Vitamin E has many roles as well, but it is best known as an anti-oxidant. Some people call it the anti-aging vitamin. Vitamin K, on the other hand, is important in blood clotting and wound healing.

These vitamins can be obtained from animal and plant sources. The vitamins derived from animal fats are much more bioavailable and thus better sources. For example, animal liver is a good source of vitamin A. Cod liver oil is beneficial as well because it contains retinol, a form of vitamin A that is most readily used by the body. Carrots, on the other hand, contain beta-carotene. Beta-carotene is vegetable vitamin A and needs to be converted to retinol in the body. Infants cannot make this conversion and children do so poorly. As a result, saturated fat from animals (e.g. butter or liver) is especially important for young children.

Some adults, such as diabetics, also have difficulty converting carotene to retinol. For these individuals, low-fat foods are not smart nutrition options. Saturated fats are also the single most important source of energy for humans. We have been educated to think of carbohydrates as the only energy-giving food, but fat is actually a more efficient energy source. This is why many primitive people have been able to thrive and have boundless energy with little to no carbohydrates in their diet.

Clearly, it's important to eat saturated fats if you want your body to function correctly. Fat, in my opinion, is the single most important part of the diet. Avoiding it can only be detrimental to your health.

Chapter 5 - Sugar Is Toxic

By the term 'sugar,' I am referring to ordinary table sugar—the substance you add to tea or coffee, and used in baking cakes and biscuits. This common sugar is also known as sucrose. When sugar is analysed in a laboratory, it is found to actually be made up of glucose and fructose in equal amounts. In fact, each glucose molecule is bound to a fructose molecule, and so these sugars exist as pairs. Table sugar is really glucose and fructose bonded together in holy matrimony. Like many husbands and wives, these two sugars are radically different from one another. You could almost say they are diametrically opposed, as one is very useful to the body while the other is very damaging.

When you eat table sugar, your body splits the bond between glucose and fructose and releases the individual sugars. The two sugars are then metabolised very differently. In truth, they should never be eaten together. They have the potential to wreak havoc on the body and cause a whole range of health problems.

Glucose is abundant in nature. It exists in many foods and is used as the main source of energy by all living creatures. Plants produce glucose during photosynthesis and this glucose is then stored as starch. Other living organisms then eat this starch as a source of nourishment. This is evidence that glucose is a very safe sugar found in natural foods that provides us with energy.

When glucose enters the bloodstream, it has certain effects on the body. One of these effects stimulates the release of insulin. Insulin escorts glucose out of the bloodstream and into the bodily cells, where the sugar cells are then broken down to release energy. The effect of insulin on fats, however, is what's really interesting. Insulin doesn't push only glucose out of the bloodstream—it also pushes fats into the cells where they are stored as triglycerides. Effectively, insulin promotes the storage of fat in the body.

Insulin Promotes the Storage of Fat in the Body

I have further placed emphasis on this statement because it shows the link between eating glucose and becoming fatter.

Fructose, on the other hand, is not commonly found in nature. It is found in fruits and honey only, and it is not used as a source of energy. Unlike glucose, fructose cannot be broken down by the majority of the cells in the body. Only liver cells have the ability to metabolise fructose. Consuming fructose destroys the liver in a manner similar to alcohol. You might say that fructose is a rather useless sugar. Even worse, it is actually very toxic—especially if it is consumed over a long period of time. Fructose is the only sugar that is known to cause damage in your body.

One of the main effects of fructose in the body is the production of fat in the liver. Fructose does not just cause a fatty liver, but also the deposition of fat everywhere in your body—in the bloodstream, arteries, abdomen, and in many organs as well. Fructose is a fat-producing sugar.

Fructose Makes You Gain Weight

Now you understand why your mother and grandmother used to say that sugar makes you fat. They were absolutely right. Fructose is converted to fat in the liver. It enters the bloodstream, and insulin then pushes it into the cells where it is stored. As a result, you become fatter and fatter. So if you are looking to store some fat in your body, eat some fructose with your glucose. The combination of these two sugars is what makes people gain weight while being unable to shift the weight. This is the root cause of the obesity crisis.

Fructose Makes the Fat

Insulin Stores the Fat

If fructose is the real cause of the obesity crisis, then where is all of this fructose coming from? Fructose is not only in fruit and table sugar, but it is in almost every processed food on your supermarket's shelves. Since the mid-1970s, it has been added to processed foods, fast foods, baby food, soft drinks, and most sports drinks. I have recently found it in gluten-free bread. In the United States during the mid-70s—where the obesity epidemic began—they replaced the fat content of many foods with high-fructose corn syrup. This corn syrup is a mixture of fructose and glucose, and it is found in many factory breads, cakes, biscuits, desserts, hamburger and hot dog buns, sauces, yoghurts, etcetera. The list is long. High-fructose corn syrup is cheap and tastes good; and so almost every food company uses it. Our exposure to fructose has increased markedly since the mid-70s.

The combination of glucose and fructose is also bad for another reason: Glycerol is needed in order to store fat in the cells as triglycerides. Glycerol is produced by splitting a glucose molecule in half. Thus, glucose assists in the storage of fats.

Glucose is harmless in any amount; fructose in small amounts is also harmless. Fructose in large amounts taken over a period of time, however, is toxic. Fructose combined with glucose and taken over a period of time is even more toxic. It constitutes as a serious toxin in need of strict control and should be removed from all foods immediately. Food manufacturers add high-fructose corn syrup to the food chain while completely understanding the consequences. Professor Yudkin's research and the research of many other scientists in the 1950s and '60s predated the addition of fructose to the food chain. These food manufacturers have committed a serious crime against humanity and should be held accountable. The government has also added to the problem by encouraging and advising people to eat more starchy foods—many of which contain high-fructose content.

Another interesting difference between fructose and glucose is the fact that fructose does not stimulate the release of the hormone leptin (or insulin for that matter). One of the ways your body knows that it has had enough to eat is by its production of leptin. This hormone tells your brain that your body has enough food so that your brain can block your hunger pangs. Glucose stimulates the release of leptin into the bloodstream, which then attaches to the appetite control centre in the brain. This gives the rest of your body the signal that you are full. Fructose does not do this. It does not stimulate the release of leptin, and you will eat tons of it without ever feeling satisfied as a result. You will feel constantly hungry and will continue to eat more, leading to a destructive and insatiable appetite.

Now you are beginning to see why sugar is so toxic. Since sugar—especially fructose—has been added to so many starchy foods, we are consuming more and more of it. Not only are we consuming more carbohydrates in our diet, but we're also generally eating more food than ever before. The quantity of food being consumed by each of us daily is increasing. Portions of food (especially in the US) have increased. There are two reasons for this: Firstly, we are not eating enough protein and saturated fat to induce a full, satisfied feeling. Secondly, the leptin hormone that tells your brain you have had enough food is not working properly. We will explore why in a bit.

We are also eating a lot of processed foods. In these foods, fat has been replaced with sugar and artificial flavouring in order to make them taste good. Fiber has been removed, which also leads to that unsatisfied feeling. This type of food will never fill you up and will lead to weight gain as a result. We are consuming particular types of carbohydrates. In the mid-70s, President Nixon wanted to make food less expensive for families on welfare. He implored the food companies to find a way to make foods more affordable to help America's low-income families. In response, food chemists developed HFCS, a sweetener that was natural and dirt-cheap. It was indeed natural, as it contained two naturally occurring sugars—glucose and fructose—and it was derived from corn, which is grown in large quantities and subsidized by the US government. HFCS became widely accessible due to the sheer abundance of genetically modified and highly produced corn.

Now let's look at why fructose does so much damage to the body in large amounts.

Dr. John Yudkin, a professor of physiology in the UK, released a book in 1971 entitled, Pure White and Deadly, which described the biochemistry of fructose in detail. He describes the serious damage that sucrose (table sugar) can do in the body, as sucrose is also a combination of glucose and fructose. Reading his book, I feel as if Yudkin was foretelling the future; everything he described has come to pass in the form of obesity, heart disease, type 2 diabetes, etc. He wrote a number of books on the topic and gave many lectures warning about the dangers of fructose. Unfortunately, the food chemists focused more on dollar signs than warning signs in their quest for cheap food.

Dr. Shafir in Jerusalem has also researched this topic and has come to the same conclusion: fructose is lipogenic (it forms fat and is dangerous in large quantities given over a period of time). Dr. Peter Mayes of Kings College, London, concurs with this statement and notes that the effects of chronic exposure to fructose worsens with time. According to Dr. Mayes's research, fructose disturbs blood cholesterol levels and leads to impaired glucose tolerance, insulin resistance. (in which insulin becomes much less effective), and then type 2 diabetes.

Dr. Richard Johnson has done a lot of experimental and clinical work on fructose and has shown that it is indeed implicated in the obesity epidemic and a host of disorders such as type 2 diabetes and hypertension. His article was published in the American Journal of Clinical

Nutrition in October 2007 and is entitled, "Potential role of sugar (fructose) in the epidemic of hypertension, obesity and the metabolic syndrome, diabetes, kidney disease and cardiovascular disease." He defines the principal role played by uric acid in the development of these disorders and suggests that the level of uric acid in the blood of an obese person can be used to predict the onset of these other disorders.

In summary, fructose has a tendency to disturb blood cholesterol levels and cause type 2 diabetes when it is consumed over a period of time. Fructose also can cause an elevation in blood pressure—a common finding in people who are overweight or obese. It can also cause a host of other disorders. Fructose is a substance more toxic than even alcohol. Nature clearly did not intend for us to consume large amounts of fructose. In nature, fructose is combined with fiber so limiting the amount you can consume, It is also combined with vitamin C which causes diarrhea if you take too much of it. This again will limit your intake. Nature has clever ways of making sure you do not consume too much of something that is potentially harmful to you.

Many people are already aware of the dangers associated with sugar and opt for artificial sweeteners because they believe them to be the safer alternative. Unfortunately, these are also damaging. I have made this same mistake by drinking diet soft drinks and thinking I was avoiding sugar. The truth about the effects of these artificial sweeteners emerged in 2012 in respected medical journals. They made it clear that substances such as aspartame and sucralose are very far from safe, and this information needs to be further and more widely shared with the general public. I have discussed this topic in my e-book, Alternatives to Sugar (London: Jemsoil Publishers, Amazon Kindle, 2013), and I have also discussed natural sugar substitutes. I have also included practical advice on how to reverse the damage done by artificial sweeteners.

Chapter 6 - Effects of High Uric Acid Levels

As you have read above, one of the consequences of metabolising a lot of fructose over a sustained period of time is an elevation in uric acid levels in the body. This has disastrous consequences as it results in a whole host of unpleasant disorders. Uric acid is notorious for causing gout, but it is rapidly becoming infamous for its role in the obesity epidemic as well. Let's see the exact effects of uric acid on one's health.

1. Blood Pressure

The pressure in your arteries is kept low by a substance called nitric oxide. Effectively, nitric oxide relaxes smooth muscle in the wall of the artery. Uric acid blocks the production of nitric oxide, which raises the tension in the wall of the artery and causes high blood pressure. It is interesting that drugs that reduce uric acid levels, such as allopurinol, lower blood pressure in obese subjects. This would suggest that treatment for high blood pressure in obese people should be reviewed.

By avoiding fructose in your diet, you can prevent the onset of high blood pressure. Do not take table sugar and avoid all processed foods, since they are the root cause of the obesity epidemic.

2. Kidney damage

High levels of uric acid can damage the kidney and lead to protein loss in the urine (proteinuria) as well as inflammation in the kidney (nephritis) and kidney stones. Other consequences of obesity, such as diabetes and raised blood pressure, can also result in kidney damage. It is important for obese patients to monitor kidney function. Ask your family doctor to do regular blood tests and ask specifically about kidney function as well as uric acid levels.

If your uric acid level is raised, it absolutely essential that you follow the diet suggested later in this book.

3. Metabolic Syndrome

Metabolic syndrome is a term used to cover the wide range of disorders suffered by obese people. It includes type 2 diabetes, heart disease, high blood pressure, abnormal blood cholesterol levels, and a fatty liver. High uric acid levels are now thought to be responsible for the onset of metabolic syndrome. According to research done in both laboratory animals and humans, high uric acid levels appear to be the common factor in the development of all of these disorders. In the 1950s, experiments on laboratory rats revealed that a high sucrose diet led to the onset of obesity, raised blood glucose levels, raised blood pressure, and abnormal blood lipid levels. However, if the rats were fed glucose alone, these disorders did not manifest; rats who were fed with fructose were the only test subjects who developed these disorders. You can see that the damaging effects of fructose have been known for half a century. You can also see clearly how differently the body handles these two sugars and how toxic fructose can be.

Fructose has been shown to produce very similar effects in humans. There is now a wealth of data available that supports its role in the development of obesity. Fructose also disturbs fat levels in the bloodstream and raises blood pressure. It results in fat accumulation in the liver (fatty liver) and within the abdomen (big belly). It also leads to abnormal blood glucose levels, insulin resistance, and type 2 diabetes. Insulin resistance was initially thought to be a consequence of obesity, but new research suggests that uric acid may be playing a key role in this disorder. Uric acid levels are now considered to be an important piece to predicting who will go on to develop metabolic syndrome.

Chapter 7 - Effects of Fructose on the Brain

Sugar is addictive. Many of us know this already from having eaten it over the years. I lived in the countryside in Northern Ireland as a child and would spend a lot of time in the local shop during weekends and holidays. I used to help out by filling bags of tea and sugar and by serving customers. I was paid in sweets such as spangles, fruit gums, pastilles, etc. My favourite time of day was when the bakery van arrived with cakes and buns, many of which were covered in icing. Working in that shop was like being in heaven—a sweet, sugary heaven. I became addicted to sweets over the months that I worked there and suffered serious health problems as a consequence. For many years I had to avoid all forms of sugar; today, I only consume small amounts very occasionally. I understand very well how difficult it is to get off sugar, and stay off it.

Experiments with laboratory rats have shown that rats, like humans, also become addicted to sucrose. They display patterns of bingeing when exposed to it and withdrawal cravings when off of it. These experiments also revealed changes in the rats' brain chemistry when given sucrose, particularly in their levels of dopamine. This alteration in brain chemistry may explain the symptoms people experience when addicted to sugar (such as depression, anxiety, and irritability).

There appears to be a link between obesity and addiction to food. Research done in the US during the early 2000s has shown that brain PET scans (similar to CAT scans) performed on drug addicts showed the same abnormalities as PET scans performed on obese people. Both sets of PET scans showed a significant reduction in dopamine receptors in certain parts of the brain. This can explain the binge-eating pattern seen in obese people. So, sugar is addictive and obese people show addictive behavioral patterns and patterns in the brain that is suggestive of addiction. There is growing evidence that obesity is a new addiction to certain foods. However, more work needs to be done to establish a link between obesity and an addiction to fructose in particular.

Interesting revelations about the damage that fructose can have on the brain were discovered more recently in 2012. An article appeared in the Journal of Physiology in May 2012 that linked fructose with disturbances in mental function.

This study was carried out by researchers in UCLA's David Geffen School of Medicine where they used laboratory rats to find out the effects of a high fructose diet on learning, memory, and problem solving. Head researcher Professor Fernando Gomez-Pinilla explained, "Eating a high fructose diet over the long term alters the brain's ability to learn and remember information. Interestingly, the researchers also found that omega 3 oils, which are known to have a positive effect on mental function, appear to reduce the negative effects of fructose."

Professor Gomez-Pinilla and his colleague, Rahul Agrawal, used HFCS in their experiment. HFCS, as you know by now, is a constituent of processed foods such as sodas, cakes, cookies, sauces, breads, etc. The average American consumes more than forty pounds of HFCS each year. The researchers trained a group of rats in a complex maze twice daily for five days. After that, they split the rats into two groups. The first group received only water and HFCS to eat, while the second group received HFCS plus omega 3 oil and water as well. After six weeks on this diet, the rats were re-introduced to the maze. The first group had a difficult time recalling the maze's path and was slower at problem solving. The second group fared much better. Professor Gomez-Pinilla suggested that HFCS is bad for the brain in the same way that it is harmful to the body.

This is further evidence of the damage that fructose in large quantities can have. If children are consuming significant amounts of fructose on a daily basis, not only is their BMI being affected, but their ability to do schoolwork and perform well in exams is too. It's time to take stock and monitor the amount of fructose that is being consumed in your and your family's diets.

Chapter 8 - Fructose is Dangerous

Nature intended us to eat small amounts of fructose—not large amounts of HFCS and table sugar. These manmade forms of sugar are causing problems at many levels in our society. Because of large amounts of fructose being consumed today—especially in the last thirty years—we are suffering physically, emotionally, and mentally. Worse still, we are now faced with a massive public health issue of obesity and metabolic syndrome. This epidemic has the ability to cripple our health service and our future, as the next generation is being affected too. We are slowly creating food addicts who will need expensive medical services and, of course, drugs to help.

I would describe fructose as a true weapon of mass destruction, one that I'm sure there would be no difficulty finding in Iraq. There is no need to worry about being attacked by terrorists with imaginary weapons when the food chemists are doing such a great job of destroying the lives of men, women, and children here at home. We have our governments, health services, dieticians, etc., all happily cooperating and reinforcing dietary advice that is blatantly wrong. If we have known about the dangers of fructose and the combination of glucose and fructose since the 1950s, then nobody can plead ignorance. I suggest that the scientific advisors, medical advisors, and food chemists be held accountable for this epidemic. If I can dig out this information in only a few weeks of research, how did this epidemic develop over a thirty-year period with not a whisper from anyone in authority? I smell a rat—and not one from the research laboratory.

The metabolisms of fructose and alcohol are almost identical. Both are metabolised mostly by the liver, and both in high amounts over a period of time are liver toxic. Acute exposure to alcohol affects the brain, which causes a drunken feeling; acute exposure to fructose does not do this, as it's not absorbed into the brain. However, chronic exposure to both can cause very similar symptoms because both are taken up by the liver and processed in the same way. Both are lipogenic (they form fat), both increase abdominal fat (beer belly), and both alter blood cholesterol levels adversely. Both cause fatty liver, both are addictive, both affect the heart (albeit in different ways), and most importantly, both affect the baby in the womb during pregnancy.

Look at the table below and compare the symptoms of chronic exposure to alcohol and fructose:

Effects of Chronic Alcohol Exposure	Effects of Chronic Fructose Exposure
Obesity	Obesity
Liver inflammation	Liver inflammation
Addicting	Addicting
Pancreatic Inflammation	Pancreas not affected
Increased Blood LDL	Increased Blood LDL
Cardiomyopathy	No Cardiomyopathy
High blood pressure	High blood pressure
Fetal Alcohol Syndrome	Fetal Insulin Resistance

As you can see, it's best to think twice before feeding your baby or young children with food containing fructose. Also, it is best to avoid fructose if you are pregnant. Essentially, HFCS and sucrose are like alcohol without that drunken feeling.

To reinforce this point, Fig 8.2 has the list of ingredients of an infant formula called Similac. It contains 43.2% corn syrup solids and 10.3% sucrose. A can of Coca Cola has 10.5% sucrose. This is what food manufacturers suggest you feed your baby, and the governments deem it as safe? How is this possible? Evidence suggests that the earlier you expose a child to sugar, the more they will crave it later on. Sucrose's effect on brain chemistry may lead to behavioral changes in children. One of the first things that I do to treat any child with behavioral difficulties is to take them off all processed foods—especially all sugars. According to a report in 2006 by Dr. Kim in the journal, Obesity, we now have an epidemic of obesity in six-month-old infants. With milk formulae like the one mentioned above, this is not really so surprising. I cannot believe that it has been allowed to get to this stage.

Fig 8.2
Ingredients of the Infant Formula Isomil (Similac)
43.2% Corn Syrup Solids
14.5% Soya Protein Isolate
11.5% Safflower Oil
10.3% Sucrose
8.4% Soya Oil
8.1% Coconut Oil

Sadly, parents are being blamed for their overweight children—as if parents are the ones supersizing their meals! Some doctors say that overfeeding should be regarded as a form of abuse or neglect. According to a report by a health correspondent for BBC News, Dr. Randell, a consultant pediatrician from Nottingham, UK, is one doctor who believes that some parents are killing their children with kindness. The Royal College of Pediatrics and Child Heath disagree and say that obesity is a public health issue and not a child protection issue.

In treating overweight children, eating a low-fat diet has no effect on the BMI at all. This is hardly surprising. As you have already learned in this book, it is not fat in the diet that is the cause of weight gain but rather carbohydrates. What does make a difference, however, is the removal of soft drinks, energy drinks, and sugary snacks from vending machines in schools. This has been tried in various locations with great success.

Obesity in children results in the same physical disorders as in adults (type 2 diabetes and the other disorders that make up the metabolic syndrome) and the same emotional problems (low self- esteem, depression, and anxiety). I find it very strange that some people blame parents for this problem. That approach displays a lot of ignorance and a total lack of sympathy. It's analogous to me prescribing you the contraceptive pill, which causes you to put on weight, and then blaming you for the resulting weight gain. How can you blame a parent of a six-month-old child for overfeeding their child? Has it not become apparent that we have an epidemic of obese infants? There is a great reluctance to look for the real cause of this epidemic. I wonder why?

There is a total lack of wisdom or common sense in the treatment of obese people. The only form of medicine that seems to be actually helping is nutritional medicine. Unfortunately, this excludes all dieticians, most of the medical profession, and virtually all of the advisory bodies set up to inform and advise politicians and public health officials. On that note, we shall now get back to that rat and explain why there is so much silence about the real cause of this epidemic.

Chapter 9 - Why the Silence?

This silence does not make sense if the negative effects of fructose—especially when combined with glucose—have been known since the 1950s and were publicised in many books, such as Professor Yudkin's in the 1960s and '70s. Fructose does not cause diabetes like glucose, so you would think that the diabetics associations worldwide would recommend fructose as a sweetener instead of glucose. Not so. They do not consider it safe for diabetics. If fructose is as dangerous and as toxic as all the researchers seem to think, then why is it not controlled by the Food Safety Authority and why are public health authorities not warning you to avoid it? Seems kind of strange!

The problem seems to be known as a "conflict of interest," otherwise referred to as "don't bite the hand that feeds you." Let me be specific. Medicine is married to pharmaceutical companies who pay for hospitals, research, medical education, medical journals, and etcetera. As a result, it would be foolish for doctors to criticise drug companies. This makes for a nice, cozy relationship.

Exactly the same type of relationship exists between food manufacturers and medical organisations, such as dietetic associations, heart associations, and nutritional advisory bodies. In most countries, dietary advice in hospitals and medical clinics in the community is provided by dieticians. The training and registration of dieticians is offered by the national association of dieticians. These associations are supposed to provide unbiased evidence-based advice to the public. Yet, they are all sponsored by private food manufacturers.

The Irish Dietetic Association is sponsored by Kellogg's, Abbott (infant cereals manufacturer), Danone, and Nutrica Medica. Pretty much the same companies sponsor the British Dietetic Association but, unlike the Irish, they refuse to reveal exactly who sponsors them. The sponsors of the American Dietetic Association are Coca Cola, Glaxo Smith Kline, Pepsi Cola, Unilever, and Kellogg's.

I have not listed all of the sponsors for each association. What would happen to these poor associations' funding if they were to tell the world that the food produced by their sponsors were making you ill and causing widespread obesity? Please note my sarcasm. These companies effectively gag these associations.

The British Nutrition Foundation is also sponsored by private companies such as Cadbury, Coca Cola, British Sugar, and Kellogg's. This is another organisation that is supposed to deliver independent scientific and medical evidence on nutrition. How can they do this when their salaries are under the control of such unethical companies?

These food companies are everywhere. For example, Flora margarine used to sponsor marathons, and they still do in some countries. They've also sponsored certain national heart associations, as in my own country. Companies such as Coca Cola also sponsor major sporting events such as the Olympics. They are well embedded in the very organisations that are supposed to collaborate with your government to make public policy. They carefully control who is allowed to speak at health conferences on nutrition—especially those dealing with obesity.

Not only are these companies making you ill, but they are also doing their utmost to make sure you never find out. It is no small wonder then that you have never heard about the negative effects of carbohydrates, but you have heard a lot about the negative effects of fats. This is called a diversionary tactic. As they focus public attention elsewhere, debate rages, and these companies get away with damaging you, your children, and society at large. These companies do not want you to hear the "wrong" message such as "sugar is bad for you" because these giant companies would effectively turn into minnows and ultimately go out of business. It is not my intention to put anyone out of business or to discredit anyone. I am merely trying to speak the truth in a free society. So, I hope you now have some idea of what lies beneath this epidemic and will be able to protect yourself and your loved ones. In the meantime, start reading labels more closely.

Chapter 10 – The Role of Emotions in Gastrointestinal Illness

Many people are aware that their emotions can determine the types of food that they eat. When stressed, angry, or anxious, for example, we attempt to quell our uncomfortable emotions with comforting foods such as sugar, chocolate, or (in some cases) starchy foods. In other words, we are eating to try to feel happier. What is perhaps not as well-known is the effect of food on our emotional state. I personally have experienced this quite powerfully.

In the past when I used to eat sugary foods, I would begin to feel irritable, anxious, and quite negative not too long afterwards. I would wake up the following morning feeling lethargic and depressed, and it was not until the afternoon that I finally began to feel a bit more like my normal self. Every time I ate sugar I received exactly the same reaction. This persisted for a long time until I finally became aware of it and then cut sugar out of my diet. Even today, I try to avoid sugar as much as possible.

If you are feeling negative about yourself and indulge in sugar or other carbs, chances are you will begin to feel worse about yourself, thus compounding the problem. This essentially sets up a vicious cycle of feeling bad, eating more comforting foods, and then feeling even worse. In order to get a handle on the problem and to improve not just your physical well-being but your emotional state as well, you must first observe the effect that different foods have on you. To observe this effect, you need to experiment with the food. Stay off of certain foods for a period of time—say one week—and then try it for a day or two until you notice the effect it has on you. Experimenting with food in this way gives you insight (and therefore power) to break this vicious cycle. If you are not sure which foods to try, just start with the ones you eat a lot, for example bread, chips, or cola.

Obesity is often associated with low self-esteem, which can result in overeating comforting foods. This is compounded by the image-conscious world we now live in, which makes it harder for overweight people to feel good about themselves. It is with this in mind that I have asked a colleague of mine to write a chapter to help you understand the importance of healing at a deeper level and to make sure you don't get caught in a vicious cycle.

Dr. Chadha has been trained as a doctor and as a psychiatrist but prefers to treat people without the use of drugs. He has been practising in Ireland for the past sixteen years and helping people with emotional difficulties. Having referred many patients to him over the years, I am confident that his holistic approach has been of enormous benefit to hundreds of people. He is a true pioneer in the field of emotional healing. He presently runs a stress reduction clinic in Blanchardstown, Dublin 15. His website is: www.brclinicstresscentre.com.

Dr. Pradeep Chadha

This chapter describes the physiology behind emotions. Emotions cause an arousal state that increases or decreases the body's demands for energy. The impact of emotional experiences stay in the body for a long time after the event has ended. Anger and fear cause an increase in the body's demand for energy. The energy demand can become chronic or persist even after the event is over. This demand results in overeating, especially on carbohydrates. These foods are the ones mainly responsible for converting into body fat, and as such, they contribute to obesity. Emotional stress needs to be addressed before a weight loss can be maintained. Without reducing this stress, the body's demands for food cannot be reduced. Therefore, weight can be lost—but not permanently. Very simple breathing exercises can help in beginning the reduction of long-term emotional stress in the body.

The gastrointestinal system forms a part of the human body. There are ten organ systems in the body:

- Sensory System

- Nervous System

- Endocrine System

- Gastrointestinal System

- Reproductive System

- Excretory System

- Respiratory System

- Skeletal System

- Circulatory System

Each of these organ systems function together and is affected by each other's system. Each organ system is made of different organs that work together as a team to achieve a particular purpose. For example, the gastrointestinal (organ) system consists of the mouth, the food pipe, the stomach, the small and large intestines, the liver, gall bladder, pancreas, and the rectum. Each of these organs is made up of tissues. Each kind of tissue consists of one kind of cell that together serves a particular function. For example, the muscular tissues in the stomach are responsible for contraction and expansion of the stomach and facilitating emptying the stomach as food moves from the stomach into the small intestine. There are other kinds of tissues in the stomach that are responsible for producing gastric acid and others that produce gastric enzymes. The purpose of the gastrointestinal system is to breakdown the food that comes into the body (digestion) and the absorption of the digested food. This absorbed food is then sent through the circulatory system to each and every part of the body.

Out of the systems mentioned above, the two that coordinate all of the systems are the nervous and the endocrine systems. Together they are referred to as the neuro-endocrine system. The sensory system (comprising of the eyes, ears, skin, tongue and nose) receives the messages from the external environment and conveys the information to the nervous system. The nervous system then instructs the endocrine system to produce various hormones in the body that quickly create the response the body needs to address a particular issue. Just imagine that this process is carrying on in your body even as you read this. The body has to be ready for any eventuality. So the body has to be alert to changes in the environment to adapt and change quickly and efficiently. If it does not do so, the body will become ill and die.

The gastrointestinal system (GIT) is also controlled by this neuro-endocrine activity. If the body is in a relaxed state, the gastrointestinal system (GIT) is easy going. It 'easily' produces juices and enzymes that digest the foods that enter the stomach, and it also easily absorbs the digested food through the small intestine. Any disturbance caused in the digestion or the absorption of food causes illness of the digestive tract.

The human body likes to function normally without any disturbances. It likes to sleep and wake up in time, do appropriate amounts of physical exercise and live in a happy environment with abundance. For the GIT to function normally, it appreciates good eating habits, which also includes eating at the right time. The body loves following a rhythm. Whenever there is a disturbance in this rhythm, the digestive system first tries to adjust to the disturbance and then if the disturbance carries on, it tends to change itself to adapt to the new change in the environment.

Disturbed sleep cycle is one condition when the GIT is disturbed. Night shifts, for example, are stressful for the body. This is because the body is then forced to work actively at a time when it is supposed to be asleep. Chronic emotional stress has a similar effect. When the body considers something as a 'threat,' it prepares itself to fight. On a short-term basis, the GIT can adapt itself to secrete the juices when the food comes into the digestive tract, even at an unusual time. But when the emotional stress becomes long-term or chronic, the GIT develops 'symptoms' of an illness.

A young man who lived alone—an immigrant—wanted help with his anxiety and depression. From the time he had migrated to Ireland, he had gained weight. He did not know the reason for this gain and he wanted to lose this weight. His history suggested that he had had been brought up in a strict environment. He came from a conservative background. This was a strain on him as he was now living in a freer society, and he wanted to enjoy his newfound freedom. The first thing that was addressed in therapy was the issue of his strict upbringing. This included addressing his anger with his parents. He maintained a daily diet diary for a few days and an interesting revelation emerged—he was consuming about 1400 calories of carbohydrates every day. This was far more than his daily requirements. He was advised to cut down on his carbohydrate intake and increase his vegetable, fruit, and protein intake; this would keep his fat intake at a normal level. Over the next four weeks, he lost about 7- 8 kilograms of weight without doing any physical exercise.

One of the exercises he was asked to do was to clasp his two hands together. He was then asked to breathe out fully and hold his breath. Then he was supposed to push his two palms together as hard as he could for as long as he could until he became breathless. He was advised to do this exercise initially three times a day for about two weeks, and then five times a day for the next ten weeks.

Emotional stress is easily bottled up. Just imagine that you are a 7-year-old child and your father has screamed at you. You don't understand that you have done anything wrong and you begin to feel frustrated and angry. Anger produces stress hormones in the body. The experience of stress may last for a minute or for a few hours. It happens again, and again, and again. You know, however, that these events last for a little while and then they eventually end. But your Unconscious mind is unable to let go of the angry energy produced each time your father gets angry with you. This tension continues to build up. Stress hormones are produced each time your father screams at you. But instead of their levels coming down and you feeling safe in his presence, you start to feel either angry or frightened of him. This fear or anger is never expressed. This buildup of tension or stress becomes what can be called an Internal Stressor.

Now when you decide to move away from home, your father may not come with you to the new place. But in your body, you carry the 'bottled up' anger that has not been expressed. When you go into a new environment, the environment challenges the body—especially the nervous system. This is experienced as physical, emotional, and mental stress. This may lead to inadequate sleep because of increased tension in the body. Then a boss or a senior colleague may speak with you rudely. It is the External Stressor affecting you now. It comes from the environment around you.

It is when the Internal Stressors and the External Stressors interact that the body experiences 'stress' or 'perceived threat'. According to the pioneering work done by Candace Pert in early 1990s, [DL25] emotional memory is stored in the body as chemicals known as tripeptides. A tripeptide consists of three amino acids that form the basis of memory blocks in the body. Each new emotional experience creates new neuropeptides that form the building blocks of emotional memories. The laying down of these memory traces is dependent on secretions and the activities of the neuro-endocrine system.

When food is consumed in excess, it cannot be digested quickly and it causes indigestion. Similarly, the body 'accumulates' the emotional effects of 'ordinary' traumatic events in life and these emotions may remain 'unprocessed.'

When emotions are aroused by traumatic experiences, they cannot be 'processed' or 'digested' quickly enough. This makes the Unconscious mind believe that the trauma is still happening. As such, the Unconscious mind has the role of making sure that you survive. So in a 'perceived threat' situation, it encourages the body to be alert and ready for an 'emergency' that it believes the body is going to face. The Unconscious mind wants to make sure that enough energy is available for you to fight or flee, so it increases the cravings for 'quick energy' foods. These foods happen to be carbohydrates, including sugars. Unfortunately for the body, carbohydrates are consumed to make more energy, even when there is no danger to the body. The Unconscious just 'perceived' a threat when there was none. Since these carbohydrates are taken in and not used up, they have to be stored somewhere or excreted from the body. The body prefers to hoard them in the form of fats. So all of the extra sugars and carbohydrates are converted to fat and stored as flab.

The Unconscious part of the nervous system is the autonomic nervous system and its connection is in the brain. Together, it controls all of the internal organs in the human body. It also includes the organs of the gastrointestinal system. The Unconscious, including the emotional part of the brain, is also responsible for our emotional experiences. It determines how the internal organs behave. If they 'believe' that you are under threat, they shut down the normal workings of the body and send the body into overdrive. This is done to ensure that the body survives. The limbic system is also linked to the nerves from our sensory organs. Changes in the environment are brought to its notice by these organs. Perception of the change as a 'threat' or a 'non threat' is made at the limbic system or Unconscious level. Even if the threat does not exist, mere perception of it prepares the autonomic nervous system to fight or flee.

This is experienced as stress. If the limbic system is already under strain due to past bottled up emotional experiences, the stage is set for the body to suffer the effects of 'perceived threat'.

The treatment of obesity consists of addressing the emotional impact of traumatic experiences along with the nutritional changes in a daily diet. Simply following a particular kind of diet or doing physical exercise to lose weight is not enough. In fact, these acts waste time and are not effective in reducing the flab. The traumatic experiences make the body seek more energy because of stress, which makes you eat more and do less physical exercise. Any weight loss regime that addresses the following three issues is likely to be more successful than others:

- Emotional trauma

- Nutrition and Diet

- Physical Exercise

Most weight loss programmes fail because emotional issues are not resolved. You may lose weight by exercise and controlling diet. But the demands of the body for food may remain the same because of the 'energy requirements' that depend on the emotional arousal state of the person.

A middle-aged overweight man had tried all kinds of weight reduction plans that included regular physical exercises. His general practitioner diagnosed him as having depression. However, he did not take the medications that were prescribed. He decided to do therapy, instead, for his personal emotional issues. It was after he had addressed these issues that he began to lose weight. Surprisingly, his weight started to decline without him making any conscious changes in his diet plan.

Before he was advised to exercise to reduce his chronic emotional stress, he was asked to scream loudly. He did it. He was then advised to do another simple breathing exercise. He was first asked to fill up his lungs with air, and then he was asked to slowly breathe out as if he was screaming in his own mind. It was recommended that he did this exercise for five minutes only, every day. This exercise helps in erasing long-term emotional tension locked up in the body. This is an 'evidence-based' technique.

The advantage of doing therapy is that the body and the mind come to a comparatively calmer state and are more accepting of life's situations.

As the restlessness and anxiety reduces in the body, it needs less energy for survival. The less the body demands energy, the less food the body needs to live on. So as the person comes to terms with life's traumatic situations, the 'craving' for food—especially energy-producing carbohydrates—reduces. As carbohydrates are consumed less than before, the body stops depositing more fat as there is no extra carbohydrate to convert to fat. In addition, the already deposited extra fat is gradually used up. So the body loses weight in a manner that is easier to maintain. The exercises given above can be done under medical supervision. This exercise is not recommended to people who suffer with cardiac problems or neurological problems like epilepsy.

   --Dr. Pradeep K. Chadha

Chapter 11 – The Treatment of Obesity

This section of the book focuses on ways to treat obesity. Treatment involves the use of diet and supplements.

In regard to dieting, one can utilize a faster method of losing weight, which involves a much stricter regime of treatment, or one can use the slower method that is less strict. The choice depends on you. The quicker method is what I always advise as it will bring noticeable results in a short time frame, which encourages you to continue with the program. However, it demands a bit more self-discipline and can be tough initially—especially during the first seven to ten days of the diet. You can always give the quick method a try and switch to the slower method if it's not for you.

Remember that there is always flexibility and there is no need to feel that you have to rigidly stick to just one diet plan. From years of experience of treating people, I can say without doubt that the initial discipline and sacrifice involved in the quick method is well worth the effort, as you will feel better more quickly and have more energy.

Here are the diet options:

Quick Method

This is in four different stages. Begin with stage one and work to stage four. The pace at which you do this will depend on your progress. This is dictated for the most part by how strictly you follow the diet plan and by how quickly your metabolic rate is, as well as by your general state of health. Generally, I perform a number of measurements on the person at the outset so that I can monitor progress objectively. These measurements would include body weight, waist circumference, body fat content, visceral fat content, and etcetera. That way, I can get a clear picture as to what is happening in the body and can then guide the person to when to change from one stage to the next. Obviously, it is impossible to do this without the person in front of me, so the purpose of this section is to give you an overview with the understanding that I cannot guide you from stage to stage.

Stage One

In stage one of the quick method, you are eliminating all forms of carbohydrates (such as starchy foods like pasta, potato, rice, bread, porridge, and cereals; as well as sugars such as table sugar (sucrose), fruit sugar (fructose), dextrose, and maltose). One is allowed to consume lactose found in milk, however. If you are diabetic and on medication, you will have to monitor your blood sugar level more closely. In stage one, one is allowed protein, fats, and oils but not carbohydrates.

Eat only the following foods in stage one:

- All red meats

- All white meats

- All fish (not in batter)

- All dairy produce

- All eggs

- All vegetables (except potatoes)

- All soups

- All salads (use olive oil and lemon juice as a dressing)

- All nuts and seeds

Please avoid beans and lentils as they will come in stage two.

Also, avoid crisp breads such as ryvita, oatcakes, and etcetera.; those will also come in stage two.

When choosing vegetables, minimise the use of root vegetables such as carrot and parsnip.

Breakfast options would include the following:

- Omelet with ham and cheese

- Yoghurt with seeds and nuts

- Bacon, sausage, and eggs

- Tea, coffee, or herbal tea

Lunch options would include the following:

- Soup and a salad

- Salad with cold meats

- Cooked meat and vegetables

- Cooked fish and vegetables

Dinner options would include the following:

- Boiled egg

- Cheese and ham

- One of the breakfast or lunch options

- Tea, coffee, or herbal tea

Stage Two

This stage involves introducing a small amount of carbohydrates into your body in the form of starch. The type of starch you digest is important, however, as you do not want to raise your blood sugar level too much. Foods that keep your blood sugar level low are called low GI (glycemic index) foods. Low GI starchy foods include brown rice, whole-wheat bran, oat bran, and whole-wheat pasta. Continue to avoid breads. You can also try adding some beans and lentils into your diet during stage two, as well as crisp breads such as ryvita (but avoid rice cakes). Also avoid commercial breakfast cereals and museli, as both will have sugars. In addition to these items, you can still eat all of the foods from stage one.

Try a little starch once a day (e.g. ryvita at breakfast or brown rice at lunch), but do not eat starch late in the day.

Stage Three

In stage three, it is possible to add in some more starchy foods to your diet. These include basmati rice, whole-wheat or rye bread, and oats, but continue to avoid all other forms of starch and all sugars. Again, only eat starch at breakfast or lunch. Continue to avoid all fruits as they contain fructose. You can also eat all of the foods from stage two.

Stage Four

In this stage you can add:

- Potatoes

- White rice

- Pasta

- Fruits

- Rice cakes

These are foods that I would use sparingly as they will raise your blood sugar significantly (excluding fruits). Best to avoid these if you are, or have been, diabetic.

Those are the four stages of the diet plan. The decision of when to move from one stage to another and which stage to begin with is best made through consultation with your doctor, nutritionist, or dietician.

The Slower Method

Stage One

This involves performing stage two of the quick method but doing so for a lot longer. In other words, you will have to avoid all forms of sugar and starch—with the exception of wholegrain rice, wholegrain pasta, a little crisp bread, and occasionally beans and lentils. Use low GI forms of starch when possible. There will be a much more gradual loss of weight with this method that will only be noticeable after a period of time, depending on your starting weight, your metabolic rate, the distribution of fat in your body, and your commitment to the diet plan.

Stage Two

This is equivalent to stage three of the quick method. Again, you will have to stay on this stage for a longer period of time.

Stage Three

This is equivalent to stage four of the quick method, and you will have to stay on this stage for a longer period of time.

Chapter 12 – Weight Loss Supplements

When buying supplements, the trick is to distinguish the useful ones from the potentially dangerous ones. There are a whole host of supplements available in the marketplace, and there is the accompanying temptation to buy some of these, especially when you read the amazing claims made by the advertisers. The truth is that most of these supplements are a waste of money and will do little to help you reduce body weight. Before purchasing any weight loss supplement, do your homework first by reading books, researching on the internet, and talking to people who have used the supplement. If possible, ask a lecturer in nutrition at a recognised university who can give you unbiased, independent advice. There is much hype and marketing claims but little hard independent scientific evidence behind most of these supplements.

When reading about the supplements below, it is important to keep in mind that carbohydrate is the problem food in your diet—not fat. However, you are probably aware of this by now by reading the previous pages. All of these supplements are available over-the-counter in pharmacies and health food shops. I will focus on the main supplements that sell best:

1. ALLI

This is an over-the-counter version of the prescription drug called Orlistat (trade name is Xenical). Alli is really a lower strength version (60mg) Orlistat. Let me first explain how it works and its side effects before commenting on its usefulness.

Alli works by reducing the absorption of fat across the gut wall; it effectively disables the enzyme lipase, which digests fat in the gut. Therefore, fat does not get digested or absorbed but is instead eliminated in the stool. It blocks about 20% of fat from being digested, which reduces the amount of fat available for absorption. It is used in combination with diet and exercise. Alli is really only recommended for people with a BMI greater than 30. It is not recommended for anyone with a BMI lower than 30, for anyone who is pregnant or breast-feeding, or for anyone with medical problems such as diabetes. The loss of weight reported with this supplement is very low. The side effects associated with taking Alli are diarrhea, urgency of defecation, flatulence, oily stools, and oily leakage from the rectum.

Comment

It is dangerous to reduce the fat content in your diet. Firstly, fat is an essential component of a healthy diet, as all cell membranes need it to function. Secondly, dietary fat is necessary for the absorption of fat-soluble vitamins such as vitamins A, D, and E. By blocking the digestion and, therefore, the absorption of fat, you are blocking the uptake of these essential vitamins—this is not a good idea. Because Alli is a drug that has to be used long-term, you are running the risk of long-term depletion of these vitamins.

The use of this drug makes very little sense. Worse still, it can cause significant harm. For example, by reducing Vitamin D intake, you are running the risk of developing osteoporosis. In my opinion, Alli is a supplement/drug to be avoided at all costs.

2. Appesat

Appesat contains an extract of seaweed that swells in the stomach and tricks you into feeling full. When you swallow Appesat, it enters the stomach, absorbs water, swells up, and stretches the wall of your stomach. Receptors in your stomach wall send signals to your brain, which turns off your hunger hormone so that you no longer feel hungry. This supplement therefore works by curbing your appetite. It is similar in action to a gastric balloon and similar to the results of a fibre-heavy diet. The manufacturers of Appesat claim that people can lose up to 5kg in three months. Appesat comes as capsules and one has to take three capsules thirty minutes before each meal. It is best taken with a lot of water. The desired effect is that one will eat smaller portions and gradually become accustomed to smaller portions in the long-term. Clinical trials suggest it is effective and safe. The Medicines and Health Products Regulatory Authority in the UK has approved Appesat. There is no need to use it long-term, as you will probably get used to eating smaller portions.

Comment

This definitely is a safe product since it is simply seaweed. It works in the same manner as extra fibre in your diet. It is, however, quite expensive at £30 for fifty capsules.

3. Bitter Orange

This supplement is the fruit of an orange tree found mainly in East Africa and tropical Asia. The Chinese used it for centuries to treat tummy problems such as nausea, indigestion, and constipation. More recently, it has been used to induce weight loss. The peel of the fruit or the dried fruit is used in tablet or capsule form to help curb weight gain.

Many weight loss supplements use bitter orange either alone or in combination with other substances. It works as a stimulant in pretty much the same way as other stimulants, such as ephedra (now banned). Bitter Orange contains a chemical called Synephrine, which speeds up the metabolic rate and in so doing, speeds up your heart rate and raises your blood pressure. By speeding up metabolism, it burns up fat reserves in the body, which leads to weight loss.

It is not recommended for anyone with a heart condition or with blood pressure problems. Also, it is not recommended if you are breast-feeding or are pregnant.

Comment

Bitter Orange does result in some weight loss, but my advice is to avoid it because it has dangerous side effects.

4. Chitosan

This rather novel substance is known to bind to fats, oils, and toxic chemicals, and to clot blood. It is presently the subject of much medical research. It is made from the shells of shrimp, crab, and other shellfish. The shells of these sea creatures are composed of chitin. The shells are crushed and made into a powder. This powder is used in agriculture, in water purification, and in wine making. Because it is so effective at soaking up fats and oils (it can absorb up to ten times its weight), it has been tested in clinical trials and is shown to be effective in absorbing dietary fats. However, the amount of dietary fat removed by Chitosan is not very significant

Comment

Again this product focuses on the reduction of fat in the diet, which is not the issue. It is dangerous to reduce dietary fat as I have explained above. I wouldn't recommend this supplement.

5. Chromium

This is a trace element needed by the body to function effectively. How it works in the body is not currently known, but it is thought to enhance the action of insulin, and by doing so, keeps your blood sugar level stable. Meats and whole grains are high in chromium; foods high in sugar are low in chromium. Since your body needs small amounts, only a tiny percentage is actually absorbed from foods. It is thought that the recommended daily allowance is 50 – 200 micrograms.

Your body is likely to be low in chromium if you eat a high sugar diet or if you are pregnant, breast-feeding, stressed, or exercising extensively. Because it has a stabilising effect on blood sugar levels, it may also help people with diabetes. However, studies done were inconclusive because the number of people tested was quite low.

Claims have been made that chromium reduces body fat and increases muscle mass. Some clinical studies do show a weight loss effect, but the results were inconclusive as only a small number of subjects were used and for too short a period of time.

Comment

It is generally not advisable to use any mineral on its own; it is better to use it as part of a multi-mineral supplement. Since we are unsure about how chromium actually works in the body, it is best not to take it— especially since studies have been inconclusive. Chromium also has side effects such as mood changes and headaches. I would not recommend it.

6. Conjugated Linoleic Acid (CLA)

This supplement is often referred to as CLA. It is a natural oil found in the produce of grass-fed animals such as lamb, sheep, and cattle. Mutton, lamb, beef, and dairy produce are rich in CLA— provided the animals were fed on fresh grass and not silage or hay combined with grain feed. CLA was originally discovered to be an anti-cancer substance as it had shown anti-cancer properties in experiments done on laboratory animals. It was later shown to be of benefit in weight loss. Thirty-five clinical trials have shown modest benefits in weight loss treatment at a dosage of 3.2 grams per day. At this dosage, weight loss amounted to approximately one pound every five weeks. Higher dosages had no additional benefits. There is definite evidence of a modest weight loss by using this substance.

More recent studies in laboratory animals report that mice treated with CLA show a rapid loss of weight. As is common with rapid weight loss, however, there is an increase in fat deposits in the liver. A fatty liver increases the risk of insulin resistance and ultimately diabetes. However, rats treated with CLA did not show significant weight loss or a fatty liver. As you can see, there is conflicting experimental evidence.

Comment

CLA does seem to benefit weight loss treatment, albeit the amount of weight lost is modest. Because CLA also has been proven with anti-cancer properties, it is a substance well worth using. Personally, I would recommend consuming meat from a butcher who has his/her own farm and who can guarantee that the animals are fed on natural pastures. Alternatively, eat organic dairy and organic meat products. If you do lose weight rapidly, it is best to check your blood sugar levels regularly as there is always the risk of developing diabetes (as mentioned above).

7. Green Tea

This is a really fascinating plant, which has been the subject of much scientific and medical research. Its health benefits are amazing and there is indeed evidence that it can assist with weight loss. Green tea is full of antioxidants that protect against degenerative diseases such as heart attacks and cancer.

The green tea plant originates in China where people drink many cups a day. The tea is made from the leaves of the plant that grows throughout China. The Latin name of the plant is Camellia sinensis. The tea is thought to protect against cancer; this may explain why the Chinese have such a low incidence of lung cancer despite the fact that they smoke so heavily.

Studies done at the University of Edinburgh reveal that green tea reduces blood pressure, cholesterol levels, body fat content, and body weight. Studies done at the Linus Pauling Institute at Oregon State University show that green tea is able to enhance the immune system and can suppress autoimmune disorders such as rheumatoid arthritis. Other medical studies have shown that green tea can improve bone density, reduce the risk of dental caries, and improve mental function.

In relation to weight loss, the tea (which is made from the leaves of the plant) does not raise your metabolic rate sufficiently to produce significant and immediate weight loss. A green tea extract in which the active ingredients are extracted and concentrated, however, has been shown to suppress appetite and speed up the metabolic rate, which burns up fat reserves. This extract has a few side effects, which include nausea, flatulence, and abdominal bloating.

In regard to preventing cancer, green tea and green tea extract have been shown to protect against different types of cancer such as breast cancer and colon cancer.

 Comment

This is a substance well worth using every day of your life. Its benefits are legendary and research supports this. For faster weight loss, use the extract (which is available in health food shops). The tea is available in most supermarkets. I would advise making a lifelong habit of drinking green tea.

8. Guar Gum

Guar gum is a natural food thickener, much like corn starch or tapioca flour. It is a much better thickener and much cheaper than corn starch. It is widely used in the food industry to thicken foods such as custard, puddings, ice cream, and etcetera. It is also commonly added to diet pills in order to induce a sense of fullness.

The FDA (Food and Drug Administration) banned Guar gum in the early 90s because when it is taken it large quantities, it can bind to liquids in the stomach and small intestine, swell in size, and block the gut. Smaller quantities, however, are quite safe to use.

Guar gum is actually a polysaccharide composed of two sugars: galactose and mannose. Research has shown that it has some useful benefits that include lowering cholesterol and increasing the absorption of calcium in the large intestine.

Comment

It is safe to use in small amounts, but it is quite ineffective as a weight loss treatment. I would not recommend using it.

9. Hoodia (Hoodia gondanii)

This is probably the best appetite and thirst suppressant in the world. The San Bushmen of southern Africa chew the leaves of this plant to reduce thirst and appetite for when they go on long hunting trips. Although it looks very much like a cactus plant, it is not. Despite this, it is commonly referred to as the South African desert cactus. The only active ingredient ever isolated from the plant is called "P57." This active ingredient was patented in 1995 by the company Phytopharm. Research done at this time indicates that it does, indeed, suppress appetite and thirst. The pharmaceutical company, Pfizer, then bought a license to manufacture P57 in pill form. To date, however, this pill has not been produced as it is still in the research and development phase. Some research indicates that it may be liver toxic. This is clearly one of the disadvantages of using isolated chemical extracts instead of the whole plant.

The fact that the plant suppresses thirst as well is of concern; reducing fluid intake can have serious consequences that include dehydration, kidney stones, loss of consciousness, and coma. It is not advisable to use hoodia if you are pregnant, breast-feeding, are diabetic, or have liver or kidney problems.

Comment

Hoodia does work by suppressing your appetite. However, it is not meant to be used continuously. The bushmen use Hoodia on rare occasions when they set off on long hunting trips. To use it daily or frequently is dangerous. Do not use it without consulting your doctor first.

10. White Bean Extract (Phaseolus vulgaris)

This is marketed as a "starch blocker." It wins the prize as best supplement because of its ability to identify the real problem food in your diet (i.e. carbohydrates). Many other supplements focus on the fat content of your diet or on appetite suppression. This is the only supplement that focuses on preventing the breakdown of carbohydrates to sugar.

White bean extract works by reducing the activity of the enzyme amylase, which digests starch in the gut. By slowing down the rate of conversion of carbohydrates to sugar, it slows down the rate at which sugar enters the bloodstream. This stabilises your blood sugar level and slows the conversion of sugar to fat in the liver.

One of the few medical studies done on white bean extract, reported in the Journal of Medical Science 2007, does indeed confirm its ability to reduce body weight, total body fat content and waist size. No long term studies have been done but it is an extremely promising substance. Safety studies also need to be done and effective dosages need to be established.

Comment

It is by far the best supplement used for weight loss. Because it stabilises the blood sugar level it is very safe and even desirable for diabetics to use. I would recommend it highly.

My Overall Advice:

Drink green tea every day, many times a day. Use green tea extract if you want to see a faster weight loss.

Use CLA daily as a supplement or eat the produce from pasture-fed animals.

Use White Bean Extract as it works and makes perfect sense.

Avoid all the other supplements.

Conclusion

I hope you've enjoyed the book and that it has been helpful to you and your loved ones. In the months and years to come you will gradually see a big shift in the types of foods we are eating. As people become more aware of nutrition, they will demand real food, organically grown food and stop purchasing processed food. Farmers will have to change their ways and reduce the use of chemicals, supermarkets will have to reduce their sale of processed food, and offer more fresh produce straight from the farm. Remember that the power lies with the consumer, not with politicians, bankers or supermarkets, and especially not with food manufacturers.

If you change your habits they will have to change theirs.

As you have learned in this book; reduce your intake of carbohydrates, eat animal fat, drink plenty green tea and take useful nutritional supplements such as a good vitamin mineral supplement plus fish oil and flaxseed oil. If you do this, not only will you lose weight, but you will also feel a lot better.

If you need any advice or help feel free to contact me. My contact details are at the beginning of the book.

I wish you all the best in your journey, be it a weight loss journey, or a search for a healthier way to live.

John Mckenna

John Mckenna was born in Newry, Northern Ireland and received a degree in Microbiology and Biochemistry from Trinity College, Dublin and a medical degree from the University of Zimbabwe. He then did numerous courses in natural medicine in Ireland, England and Austria and has spent the last twenty five years practicing natural medicine. He is the author of the international bestselling Alternatives to Antibiotics (Gill & MacMillan, 1999) and Hard to Stomach: Real Solutions to Your Digestive Problems (Gill &MacMillan, 2002) as well as several e-books. He can be followed on twitter @authorjohnmck .

Acknowledgements

Firstly, I would like to thank my daughter Jackie for all the work she has done in preparing this book for publication, and with getting it published as an e-book. She is an excellent writer, editor and publisher. I am very proud of you and love you very much.

Secondly, I would like to thank Pradeep for agreeing to help with a chapter in this book. You have been a great friend and colleague. I thank you sincerely for being such a great help to my patients and to me as well. Through your help I am able to express my emotions much more freely.

Thirdly, a huge thanks to my editor at Gill and MacMillan, Fergal Tobin, for giving me the freedom to publish this book as an e-book.

Finally, I would like to thank all my patients without whom this book would not have seen the light of day. You are the key to my success as I have learned so much from you. I appreciate your kindness and support over the years.

Bibliography

Ahrens,E.H. "Carbohydrates, Plasma Triglycerides and Coronary Heart Disease". Nutrition Reviews, 44/2 (1986), 60-64

Davies,S. And Stewart, A. , "Nutritional Medicine": Pan MacMillan, 1987

Fallon,S., "Nourishing Traditions", Washington:New trens Pub Inc., 2001

Johnson, R.J., et al..."Potential Role of Sugar (Fructose) in the Epidemic of Hypertension, Obesity and the Meatbolic Syndrome, Diabetes, Kidney Disease and Cardiovascular Disease", American Journal of Clinical Nutrition, 86/4 (October 2007), 899-906

Kendrick,M., "The Great Cholesterol Con", London: John Blake Publishers, 2007

Keys,A., "Coronary Heart Disease in Seven Countries", Circulation, 41 (supplement) (1970), 1 – 211

Lopez,A., "Some Interesting Relationships Between Dietary Carbohydrate and Serum Cholesterol", American Journal of Clinical Nutrition, 18 (1966), 149-153

Mann,G.V. et al ... "Atherosclerosis in the Masai", American Journal of Epidemiology, 95/1 (January 1972), 26-37

McKenna,J., "Alternatives to Sugar", London: Jemsoil Publishers, Amazon Kindle, 2013

McKenna,J., "Alternatives to Antibiotics", Dublin: Gill and MacMillan, 1996

McKenna,J., "Hard to Stomach", Dublin: New Leaf, 2002

Shils, M.E., et al... "Modern Nutrition in Health and Disease", Philadelphia: Lea & Febiger, 1994

Yudkin,J., "Pure, White and Deadly" (new edition), London: Penguin,2012

Printed in Germany
by Amazon Distribution
GmbH, Leipzig